I0705373

THE DNA MYTH

DEBUNKING COMMON MISCONCEPTIONS ABOUT GENETICS

50 concepts of epigenetics & essential facts about nutrition

Author; Yunus Güven
1st Edition: July 2020

Translator; Funda Gültekin-Hadjami
(email: gueltekin-hadjami@gmail.com)

This book is dedicated to
my beloved son Imraan,
my everything.

I hope that one day
you will be proud of me
and that you will take a
similar altruistic
and inquisitive path to the one
your father took

For me, your father,
knowledge is the
greatest good of all
and its application
is the path to true bliss.

"Knowledge brings the greatest yield,
more than any farmer or banker
can bring.

Only he who knows will realize,
what knowledge books can yield
with blood, sweat, and tears

It is a yield
no one can count,
But know that
knowledge is not everyone's bounty."

My son, always remember:

"Knowledge is a virtue."

Love,
Your father

"The doctor of the future will give no medication, but will interest his patients in the care of the human frame, diet and in the cause and prevention of disease."
Thomas Edison (1847-1931)

Instagram: @the.dna.myth

Enlightenment

<u>Immanuel Kant once said:</u>

"To think for oneself means seeking the highest touchstone of truth in oneself (that is, in one's reason), and the maxim of thinking for oneself at all times is enlightenment. "

The purpose of this book is to enlighten the reader about "nutrition and health". Very often, the information we receive from the mass media is distorted and underlies the interpretive sovereignty of partisan institutions. Representing complex scientific disciplines that impact every sphere of our lives, general social paradigms found in the relevant topics often invoke a feeling of helplessness, disempowering the individual unknowingly. To understand the human body, one of the most complex organisms on the planet, profound knowledge is needed in the different fields of naturopathy, physiology, psychoneuroimmunology (PNI), genetics, and epigenetics. This is why it is down to a collective group of individuals or the relevant experts to maintain a skeptical, inquisitive mindset. For this is the only way to ensure good health in reality and guarantee that we approach disease properly and spread scientifically proven teachings on health and well-being.

In a similar vein:

Enlightenment is man's leaving his self-caused immaturity. Immaturity is the incapacity to use one's intelligence without the guidance of another. Such immaturity is self-caused if it is not caused by lack of intelligence, but by lack of determination and courage to use one's intelligence without being guided by another.

Enjoy reading, everybody!

Foreword by Andrea Bachmair

I will never forget the day I met Yunus for the first time!
A patient that was due his first appointment with me
rang me up to ask whether it would be ok to bring someone
along to the appointment, someone who had a lot of
questions about vaccination and general health. I didn't
have much time that day, so I had to say no to his request.
When the patient came for his appointment, what did I see?
There was someone standing next to him in the doorway:
"So, I brought him along after all. He knows your books and
really wanted to meet you!" It was meant to be, I thought.
So be it! I quickly realized that he was very interested in
this field, and he was always asking meaningful questions.
This was the beginning of a wonderful friendship. When
Yunus is interested in something, he becomes completely
immersed in the subject and wants to know everything. He
pores over numerous textbooks and he doesn't shy away
from the less common paths – just think of how him and I
came to meet.

Anyone who has sought his counsel will know exactly what I'm talking about. He shares his knowledge and wants to help people to find their way back to good health.
This first book of his, **"The DNA Myth"**, is intended to remind people how easy it is to live a healthy life and to take a little more responsibility for yourself and your health. Nowadays, many people have stopped taking responsibility for their own health, often even taking health for granted. And when something is wrong, you simply go see a doctor.

If we don't change our unhealthy ways of living, our unhealthy diet, however, not even a doctor will be able to help us. WE are responsible for our own health!

Dear Yunus, I wish you the very best of success with your first book! I hope that your book will encourage many to pay greater attention to their health and their way of life. to take a look behind the scenes of the food and pharmaceutical industry.

Andreas Bachmair
Licensed naturopathic doctor in Kreuzlingen, Switzerland
Specialized in the treatment of vaccine-related injuries
Lecturer at various accredited alternative medicine schools in Switzerland

"The man who omits a daily investment
in his health will one day have to
sacrifice a great deal to his illness."

Sebastian Kneipp

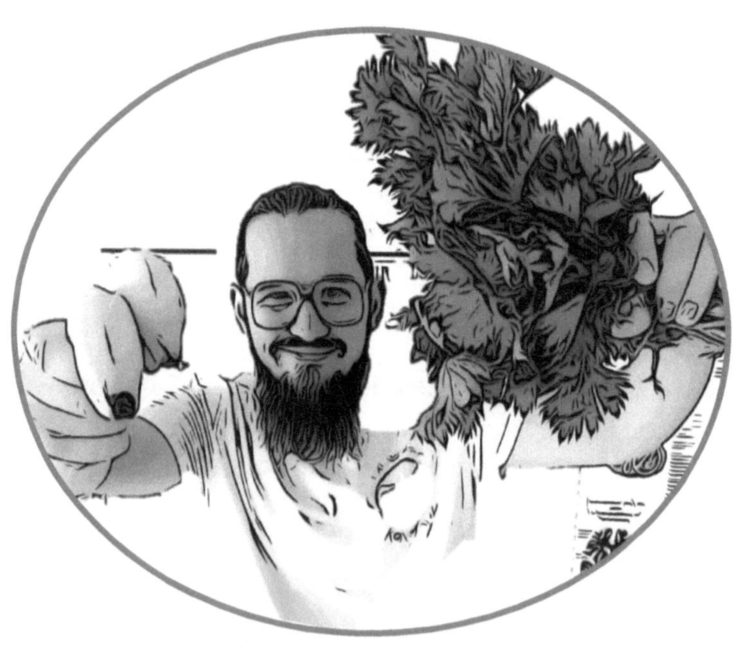

Introduction to scientific thinking and epigenetics

A saying in Germany goes:
"Today's truth will become tomorrow's lie."

You might be wondering why I've quoted this saying at the beginning of my book?

The reason Is that I want to put the following to my readers: when it comes to health, there is no such thing as **"a single truth"**.

I wish to show you that commonly held opinions on today's health and nutrition myths **are too dogmatic, too fanatic, or simply just wrong.**

Everybody claims their diet to be the one true **"Holy Grail"**, believing their way is the only way to become fit and healthy. What they forget, however, is the individual. Something that is right for one individual might be wrong for another.

Friedrich Nietzsche once said:

"There is only perspective seeing."

This statement also applies to the latest state of research in this field as well as how research findings are interpreted and evaluated. The extent to which a "health or nutritional truth" can be said to be upheld or proven depends not only on further studies that substantiate the "truth," the powers that be that interpret the findings, but also on trivial things such as the interest groups involved in the study and whoever is financing it.

The art here lies is the ability to start from a neutral standpoint and join the dots yourself, evaluating the information and reading between the lines.

As Johann Wolfgang von Goethe put it so succinctly:

"...The truth has to be repeated constantly, because error also is being preached all the time, and not just be the few, but by the multitude. In the press and encyclopedias, in schools and universities, everywhere error holds sway, feeling happy and comfortable in the knowledge of having majority on its side.

Just look how history is repeating itself today! The parallels to Goethe's time can be seen today in reference to the Internet, search engines, magazines or even today's "educational institutions". Goethe, a well-known, respected voice of authority, recognized that **truth and error** can be regarded in all manner of ways and this was his maxim when it came to the interpretation of so-called "truths".

<u>**A person's cultural background, customs, food tolerances, general state of health, mental health, and environmental influences must come into the equation when it comes to health.**</u>

In my opinion, this should be the starting point for nutritional concepts that are tailored to individual health and nutritional needs.

The somewhat bold title of my book stems from the widespread assumption that we have a genetic predisposition to disease – an assertion that is one of the greatest lies of our time.

To emphasize this once again:

"Today's truth will become tomorrow's lie."

Epigenetics is the very science that has proven this. This science shows us how environmental factors - including nutrition - affect our genes. Allow me to give you a simple example:

We have all heard the words: "Your father, his father, and his father before him had it – you'll get it, too. There's no way around it."

Yet, it is a scientific fact that changes in lifestyle and behavior affect our gene expression positively. It thus follows that recovery and healing processes can be triggered by the body.

Epigenetic Factors

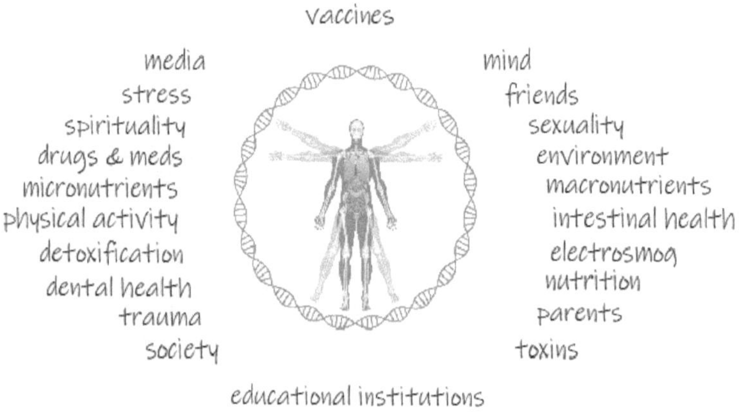

Back in his day, Arthur Schopenhauer commented:

"All truth passes through three stages.
First, it is ridiculed.
Second, it is violently opposed.
Third, it is accepted as being self-evident."

This astute statement by Arthur Schopenhauer is reflected in the lie about our genetics that is being propagated in the 21st century. In the beginning, doctors ridiculed alternative doctors and naturopaths who put forward the thesis that **genetics**, rather than being a fatalistic mechanism, can be changed for the better by our behavior and lifestyle. This idea is increasingly gaining ground in therapeutics, and thanks to medical successes, it is also being looked at as a real possibility. This is largely thanks to the Internet, a multiplicative-pluralistic platform, which has brought epigenetics to the fore. After all, behavioral and lifestyle changes have been seen to result in recovery in patients who had been condemned to suffering and inevitable death from terminal illness.

People are being deprived of their vitality not only through erroneous information and psychological manipulation tactics on the part of the relevant institutions, but also by their own subconscious mind, which is programmed to resign itself to illness.
Realizing this is the first step – developing an awareness for the habits you have developed and the resulting suffering, pain and powerlessness they have caused. Habits can destroy you but they can also be the key to the highest levels of success.

As another German saying goes:
"Your success is the sum of all your positive habits."

Once you realize this, or when the suffering becomes too much, you can gradually start to change habits and embark on the path to success and vitality.

Another problem in today's society is the false understanding of recovery. We are born into a system that teaches us nothing about disease prevention. Yet, this is the very origin of the solution to health problems.

"Prevention is better than cure!"

For centuries, this central message has been anchored in peoples' minds. Lifestyle diseases, as we know them today, did not exist before.

The importance of prevention was seen as far back as the time of Hippocrates. To loosely quote Hippocrates:

"Those who wish to stay strong, healthy and young, and prolong their lives are moderate in all things. They breathe clean air, care for their skin daily, perform physical work, keep their heads cold, their feet warm, and heal minor ailments by fasting rather than by medication."

We have since lost touch with pearls of wisdom such as these, leaving us incapacitated and with no sense of responsibility for our lives. Yet, a sense of **responsibility for oneself** is the most effective, in fact the only acceptable way – and what we ought to be striving for.

Otto Bismarck once said:

How accurate his words are! Because the moment we place our health in the hands of someone else, it will be handled either responsibly, or in line with what the system dictates – after all, it is not their health. If we are to live with a clear conscience and a full sense of responsibility, we must take responsibility for ourselves in every respect.

To use the words of Voltaire:
"We are responsible not only for what we do, but also for what we do not do."

A huge step towards changing your lifestyle and behavior for the better is to consistently follow **the nutritional principles outlined here.**

Allow me to take you on a journey. Discover a new side to nutrition that involves neither denial nor huge limitations. What's more – you will be surprised about the variety of food and all the possibilities that will help greatly improve your well-being and boost your vitality.

The Two Golden Rules

1. "Let food be thy medicine and thy medicine be thy food."
Hippocrates

2. "The dose makes the poison."
Paracelsus

These two principles form the basis of my book, which is devoted to the universal laws of nutritional anthropology. From the beginning of human existence, our health and sickness have been subjected to the negative or the positive effects of our diet.

This book is based on ten years of experience as a health and nutrition consultant, self-taught knowledge of alternative medicine, and the latest scientific research findings.

Whether individuals or groups, those who fail to follow these basic laws of the body will sooner or later suffer the loss of vitality or health.

It can thus be seen as a central theme that runs through the jungle of nutrition myths. My love for hard facts has played the biggest role in making my book a reality, yet it is mere wishful thinking to believe that this book is flawless. It is with great humility that I maintain an open mind to new findings, which will be incorporated into future editions of the book. For the greatest obstacle to knowledge is ignorance.

Chronic diseases are diet-related. We have eaten ourselves into this mess and now we have to eat ourselves back out.
Mark Hyman

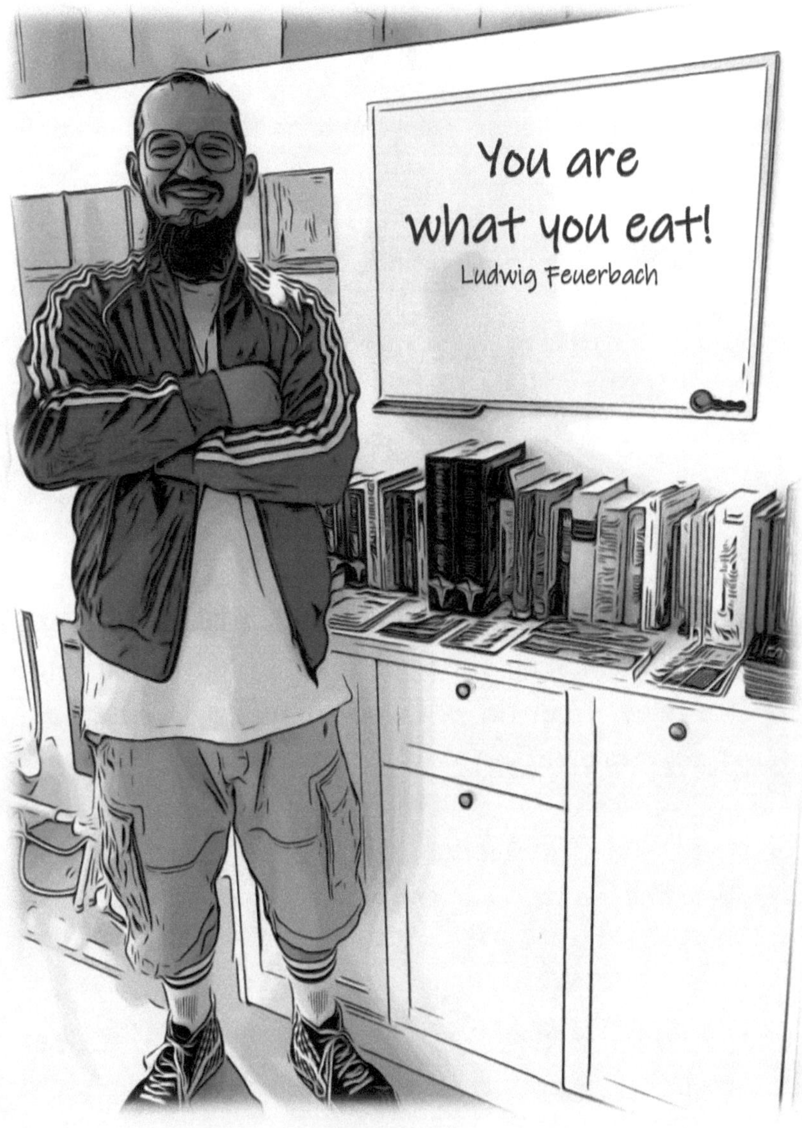
You are
what you eat!
Ludwig Feuerbach

1.

"Death dwells in the intestines!"
Socrates

Even centuries ago, people knew that diseases more often than not begin in the intestine. The greatest burden on our body comes from the things we allow to enter our body and the disease-promoting habits we cling to.

Dr. Pierre Dukan said:
For the first 50 years of your life, the food industry is trying to make you fat with their sugary and fatty products. Then, the second 50 years, the pharmaceutical industry is treating you for everything.

2.

One of the most renowned nutritionists, Dr. med. Bruker (1909 - 2001), said: "80 percent of all diseases are preventable, diet-related lifestyle diseases."

In other words: The food you eat will either makes you sick or fit and healthy. If you take drugs, you will quickly realize how bad they are for you.
An unhealthy diet is also a drug. Slowly but surely it will kill you.

3.

Learn to be hungry!
"Sirtuin" is an energy-saving gene that is activated when you fast. This gene extracts and stores as much energy for your body as possible from as little food as possible.
The minute your hunger activates this gene, damaged cells in your body are located and repaired.

Did you know that 9 million people die every year from undernourishment, while three times as many people die from supernutrition?
The 4 best known lifestyle diseases – cancer, cardiovascular diseases, strokes, and diabetes – are the outcome of the suppression of this particular gene as well as overeating.

Tip: A plant-rich diet can also activate this gene, just like fasting does. But how? Because it contains a lot of polyphenols (plant secondary metabolites) that trigger gene expression to activate Sirtuin.

4.

Fasting or intermittent fasting allows you to gain control over your body and adjust your hormonal balance. This in turn will regulate your **hunger and satiety hormones.**

You should fast for at least 12 – 18 hours and eat over a period of 6 hours a day. BTW: Moderate coffee consumption has a positive effect on the body, as coffee contains valuable secondary metabolites, although only quality organic coffee is recommended. Stay away from the poison that is conventional coffee.

Note: High-protein foods are satiating.
A combination of high-protein foods and fiber regulates your blood sugar and makes you feel satiated for longer. Plus, fiber supports the most important organ in your body - your intestines. Ideally, your food should come from plant sources. For excessive consumption of animal protein has been proven to make you even more sick or decrease your vitality, especially with those in poor health or suffering from a chronic illness.

High-fiber/high-protein sources

- Sweet lupine
- Soybeans
- Soybean sprouts
- Natto
- Quinoa
- Buckwheat flakes
- Paleo muesli
- Chia pudding
- Chia seeds
- Lentils
- Chickpeas
- Hemp seeds
- Peas
- Mung beans
- Rice protein
- Pea protein
- Gluten-free/cereal-grain-free bread
- Coconut or rice noodles
- Hemp protein
- Soy protein
- Pumpkin seed protein
- Carob germ protein
- Sprout protein powder
- Vegetable spaghetti
- Shirataki noodles
- Konjac noodles
- Rice noodles
- Lentil noodles
- Chickpea noodles
- Hummus
- Teff pasta
- Buckwheat noodles
- Corn/sweet potato noodles

These sources of protein can be bought as shakes in organic food stores or online. The shakes can be used to create delicious smoothies or can be incorporated into your meals. Protein powder is a simple, convenient, and quick way to cover your daily protein needs. Protein is good for connective tissue, it helps build muscle, it strengthens the immune system, balances hormones, and helps you sleep.

5.

"Toxic hunger" is a feeling of hunger that comes from your **mouth.**
When you see mouthwatering ads on TV, you immediately feel hungry, even though you have just eaten. **BUT,** your body is tricking you! So question this feeling and teach your body to feel **true hunger.**

6.

"True hunger" is a feeling that comes from your stomach when your tummy growls or you have slight "hunger pangs" in the stomach area. If you can read your body's signals properly, you will notice when your energy levels and blood sugar start to drop and when it is time to eat.

7.

Make it yourself!
Junk food and fast food are
bad for your health and will
make you tired.
I say: "Fast food will make you
happy for a minute but being
healthy will make you happy for
a lifetime."

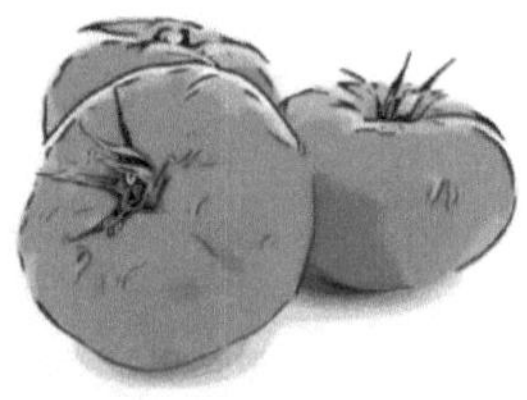

8.

Plan your meals
one day in advance.

Don't let your diet become
your religion! Make the
change yourself and **leave
others be** unless they are
genuinely interested.

9.

Avoid the bakery when you're on the go!

Wheat products are addictive and low in nutrients. They only satiate for a short time and cause inflammation in the intestines. **Gliadin,** a protein found in wheat, releases exorphins which have the same effect as opium. These exorphins pass through the blood-brain barrier and are bound to opioid receptors, triggering an addiction to wheat. This is particularly the case with the types of wheat we have nowadays. **Stay away from them!** There are so many other yummy foods out there... you just have to discover your love for them.

10.

Always take a healthy snack
with you when you're on the go!
This could be nuts, veggies, fruit,
rice cakes, dates, berries, or
dairy-free chocolate with a high
cocoa content
(min. of 80 %).

Berries should always be part of your diet. Berries contain high levels of phytochemicals that display anti-inflammatory properties, can help lower the risk of cancer, and are rich in vitamins and minerals, too!

Raspberries - Blueberries - Strawberries - Blackberries - Acai berries - Cranberries - Goji berries - Mulberries

11.

Don't go grocery shopping when you're hungry!
Otherwise, your shopping cart will soon be filled with unhealthy, high-calorie junk food.

12.

Make a shopping list
before you go to the grocery
store – and stick to it!
**Stay strong and restrain
yourself!**

13.

Listen to your body and pay attention to the signals your body sends after you've eaten – your body will tell you **what is good for you and what is not.**

Lucretius (c. 96 – c. 54 BC) said: "One man's meat is another man's poison."

14.

Try to buy food that doesn't
have a long **list of ingredients**,
unless they are wholesome or
good for you, of course.

15.

whatever you buy, try to buy
organic – preferably from
certified organic labels.

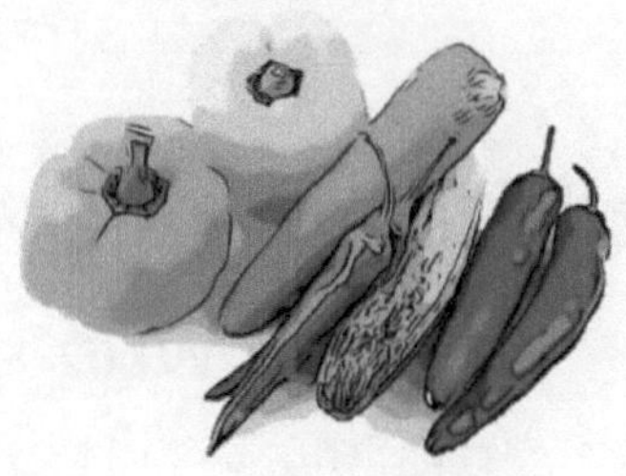

16.

Buying organic food may be more expensive in the short term, but it will pay off in the long run. If you were to get sick from unstable gut flora or carcinogenic pesticides, you would be willing to pay any price just to regain your heathy. So every penny you spend on organic food is in fact an investment in your own body.

"Tell me what you eat, and I'll tell you who you are!"
Jean Anthelme Brillat-Savarin (French author, 1755-1826)

The Environmental Working Group (EWG) publishes an annual list of the "dirtiest" conventional produce. i.e., produce with the highest pesticide residue concentrations.

EWG's Dirty Dozen for 2020:

- Strawberries
- Spinach
- Kale
- Nectarines
- Apples
- Grapes
- Peaches
- Cherries
- Pears
- Tomatoes
- Celery
- Potatoes

EWG's 2020 Clean Fifteen:

- Avocado
- Sweetcorn
- Pineapple
- Onions
- Papaya
- Peas
- Eggplant
- Asparagus
- Cauliflower
- Cantaloupe Melon
- Broccoli
- Mushrooms
- Cabbage
- Honeydew Melon
- Kiwi

N.B.: The EWG updates this list every year:

17.

Drink natural spring water
and steer clear of tap water!
It is contaminated with drug
residues and traces of hormones.
If you do drink tap water,
always use activated carbon
filters. Drinking reverse osmosis
water occasionally can also help
your rid your body of toxins.

More than half of your body is made up of water. If you drink too little, your blood will thicken, and your kidneys won't be able to remove toxins from your body properly. Try to drink at least 6 – 8 cups of water daily (8 – 10 cups if you work out). Water suppresses your appetite, aids the detoxification process, and boosts your metabolism.

18.

Avoid wheat products! They damage the valuable gut flora (which make up 80 percent of your immune system), **make you addicted, make you feel sluggish and tired, and are very low in nutrients.** Cereal grains (wheat, oats, spelt, rye, couscous, bulgur, etc.) contain anti-nutrient compounds such as **gluten, lectin and phytic acid,** which cause imbalances in gut flora, ultimately leading to Leaky Gut Syndrome and malabsorption.

Phytic acid decreases the body's ability to absorb minerals such as calcium, magnesium, iron, and zinc. Essential digestive enzymes such as pepsin and trypsin are also blocked, promoting candida overgrowth in the intestine.

Cereal grains should be avoided altogether if you are sick or suffering from chronic fatigue syndrome.

Alternative foods

Gluten-free foods	Gluten-containing foods
Buckwheat	Durum wheat
Amaranth	Spelt
Beans	Single-grain wheat
Nut flour (almond flour)	Graham flour
Arrowroot flour (Maranta)	Flatbread / pita bread
Gari (Manioc flour)	Barley
Sweetcorn	Semolina
Bean flour	Oat flakes, oat milk, oat flour
Millet	Industrially produced soy imitation
Millet flour	products (typically contains wheat flour)
Potato flour	Khorasian wheat
Tapioca	Couscous
Chickpeas	Malt
Flaxseeds	Wheat (bran, germ, starch)
Corn flour	Matzo flour
Quinoa	Orzo (type of pasta; Italian for barley)
Rice (of all types)	Rye
Teff flour	Seitan (wheat meat)
Rice bran	Tofu (often contains gluten or gluten
Sago	flour)
Soy flour	Emmer
Sweet potato	Triticale (a cross between wheat and
Grain-free, gluten-free bread	rye)
(which most stores now stock)	Bulgur

19.

Food choices are important.
When you go grocery shopping,
always choose food with the
lowest glycemic load. **Low GI
foods put less stress on your
pancreas and your body.**
GI charts can easily be found
online.

20.

Pasta and bread dull your mind **and** make you lethargic. Your intestines are often called your second brain – and wheat products can cause a lot of damage to the intestines. You have more nerve strands in your intestines than you have in your brain. If we look at embryology, we see that the brain starts to develop from the intestines. This shows us the importance of the intestines.

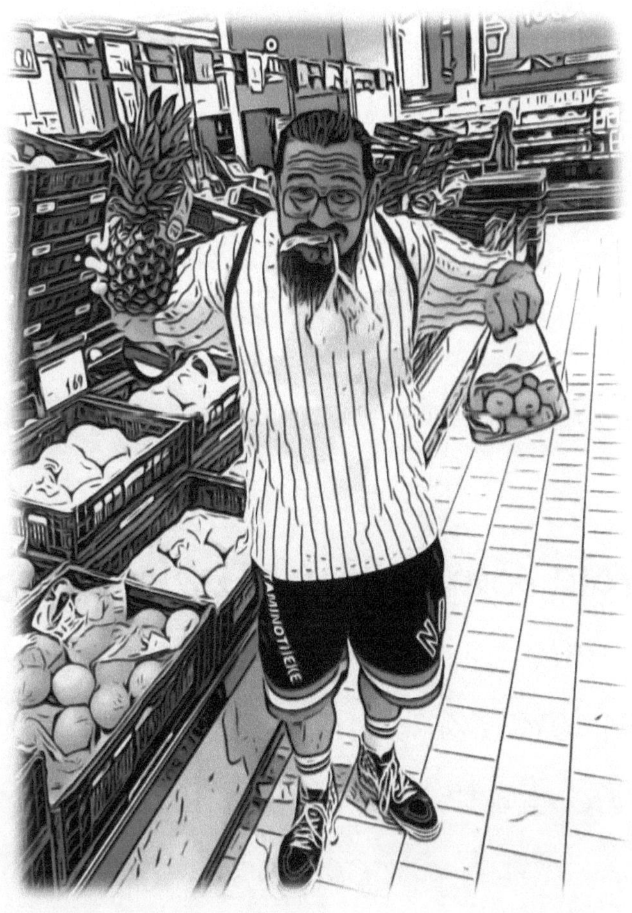

In the first half of our lives, we sacrifice our health to earn money; in the second half of our lives we sacrifice our money to regain our health. And during all that time, both our health and our time will have dwindled.

Voltaire

21.

Avoid conventional baked goods. If you fancy a snack, make your own low-carb or paleo desserts - the Internet is full of great recipes.

22.

Try your best to avoid processed and refined food. They are the curse of the 21st century and contribute to all lifestyle diseases.

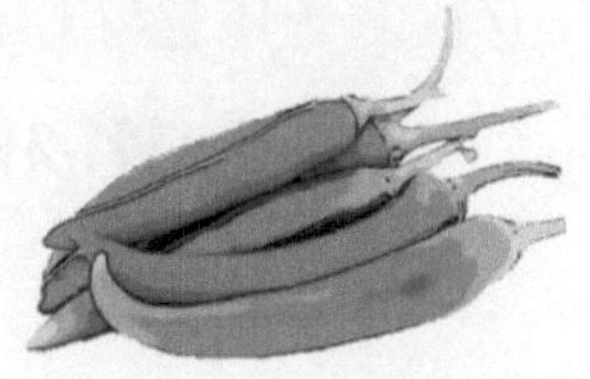

23.

Do your best to avoid high GI, processed carbs **such as pizza, pasta, fries, and bread.** Instead, go for alternatives or pseudograins such as **quinoa, amaranth, and buckwheat.** Other great alternatives are millet, rice, manioc (tapioca), and sweet potatoes.

Pseudograins...

are foods that resemble grains and can be used in the same
way as grains, even though, biologically speaking, they do
not belong to the family of cereal grains. The seeds are
usually very rich in complex carbohydrates, protein, minerals,
trace elements, and healthy fatty acids.

Pseudograins, while not your typical baking grains like
wheat or rye, can be used in a similar way to common types
of grains.

The most important pseudograins:

- Buckwheat - knotweed family
- Quinoa - foxtail family
- Amaranth - foxtail family

24.

Avoid conventional dairy products!
If consumed regularly, they can trigger allergic reactions and promote acne, pimples, skin blemishes, inflammation, or autoimmune diseases.
Dairy cattle reared on intensive cattle farms are **artificially inseminated, and neither pasture-raised nor pasture-fed. They live high-stress lives,** pumped full of drugs, antibiotics, and steroids.

25.

Conventional dairy products can **destroy your intestines.** Healthy gut flora is VITAL for optimal health. Factory farmed milk is high in omega-6 and omega-9 fatty acids, which can cause inflammation. **After pasteurization and homogenization, factory farmed milk is no longer wholesome or good for your health.** This also applies to pasteurized and homogenized organic milk unless it is **organic raw milk.**

Dairy substitutes

Substitutes for dairy products	Dairy products
Soy milk Almond milk Rice milk Almond rice milk Millet milk Coconut milk Cashew milk Hazelnut milk Macadamia milk Cream of rice, coconut cream, soy cream Plant-based yogurt (coconut, almond, lupine) Coconut oil Vegan cheese products (with as few additives as possible) Optionally: raw dairy products (only if you can digest these products; if not, they are best avoided)	Milk Cream Yogurt Butter Cheese

26.

Ethically farmed, raw organic milk and dairy products may be consumed in moderation. In fact, consumed occasionally, raw organic milk is a rich source of nutrition. This kind of milk is only recommended, however, if you can digest it properly. If you suffer from a chronic illness or chronic pain, drinking milk will only exacerbate it, which is why it should be avoided altogether.

27.

Sugar is poison!
Cancer cells consume **200 times more sugar than healthy cells.** This effect was discovered by Nobel Laureate Otto Warburg in the 1920s (the Warburg effect). The consumption of sugary foods is one of the biggest causes of cancer, it destroys your teeth, and blocks the arteries. **Food** containing sugar is breeding ground for yeast that will impair your gut flora. Certain intestinal bacteria will overgrow, blocking energy production and reducing the gut's ability to absorb nutrients.

An average person who eats large amounts of processed carbs for breakfast, lunch, and dinner as well as between meals **will produce as much insulin in one day as someone living a few hundred years ago would have over their entire life.**

Ultimately, you will become diabetic. You will develop type 2 diabetes, as your cells become insulin resistant. The sugar in the blood no longer enters the body's cells, causing the body to produce more and more insulin. The result is a vicious circle!

Many people don't know that sugar can also cause long-term damage to your brain.
Excessive sugar consumption and excess insulin production affect the function of the insulin receptors in the cells, making them resistant to sugar. The brain forgets how to use sugar as a source of energy. The sugar/glucose deficiency in the cells means that the neurotransmitters which are important for brain function can no longer be produced sufficiently. This has a lasting impact on brain function and can lead to neurodegenerative diseases such as Alzheimer's and dementia. This is also called type 3 diabetes. Moreover, too much insulin suppresses the health-enhancing synthesis between growth hormones and melatonin, the hormone that regulates our sleep/wake cycle.

28.

Avoid refined sugar and use alternatives such as xylitol, erythritol, or a good raw organic honey.

29.

Try to keep your diet as vegan/vegetarian as possible and eat as much raw food as you can. **The benefits of a predominantly plant-based diet (with very little meat) speak for themselves.** Indigenous people such as the inhabitants of the Japanese Okinawa Islands and the Tsimané, for example, are vegans, vegetarians or consume very little meat. They are some of the healthiest people on earth. The Mediterranean diet has also proven to be very healthy. Studies show these types of diets to have the greatest health benefits.

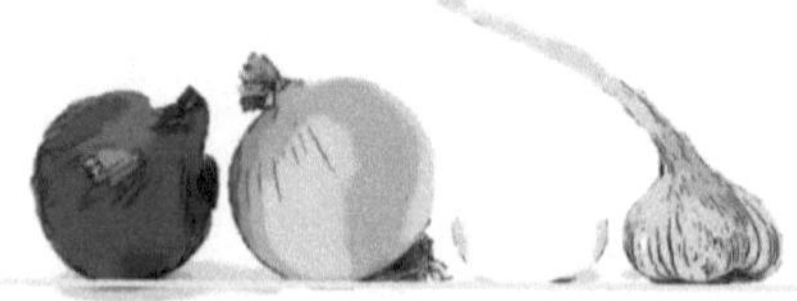

"Divide et impera" - *"Divide and rule"*
"Panem et circenses" - *"Bread and circuses"*

To all the meat eaters and vegans out there: It is not about dividing the people and trying to win diet and nutrition battles with **"pseudo-arguments,"** turning your diet of choice into an ideology or religion of sorts without even realizing it. People are divided enough already! What we need is more peace and respect for one another! Moreover, we need to make the transition to more sustainable living to protect our planet! Teach by example, clarifying only where clarification is needed to help reduce the damage done to fellow human beings, wildlife, and nature. **Don't fall for institutional divides or the perfidious attempts of the media to divide people. Centuries ago, the Roman Empire used these very methods to distract the masses, leaving them to rot in their proletariat lives.** Join hands, come together to make the world a better place, and don't get caught up in endless discussions over whether eating meat is healthy/unethical or not or whether a plant-based diet is insufficient/unethical or not. This will get you nowhere fast!

Looking at it from a neutral perspective, these attempts at conversion, as in vain as they are, are in line with an understanding of governing shaped by Imperial Rome: **"Give them bread and circuses!"** In the past, the rulers organized primitive games at which their "favorites" killed each other in bloodthirsty battles! And the citizens regarded this as their leisure activity. Nowadays, people are pushed into ideological battles with each other with "bread and circuses," detracting from the real problems we have on our planet, leaving the non-collective interests of the true evildoers on the planet undiscovered. **Don't turn your diet into the maxim of all of your actions.** Let it be everyone's own business what they eat, which is not to say you may not pass on any wise advice if and when the situation calls for it.

Clarification without ideology is the solution. This is
the only way you can achieve change or makes
things better. Change is a process and you need to
trigger this process in people using intelligence and
reason. This is the only way your good advice will be
heard and followed, resulting in better health, or
reducing the damage to our planet. From a
psychoanalytical point of view, human beings like to
feel a sense of moral superiority when engaged in
discussions, underpinning them with
"scientific/factual evidence" or even cultural
paradigms. Yet, this approach can never lead to
the truth. As a result, there will be no
improvement on either side. Instead, we will see
more dogged ideological struggle. Our minds are no
longer open to other opinions and views. The long
and short of this is, don't be an instrument of
division but an instrument of peace. A nice saying in
Germany goes: "When two parties fight, the third
party rejoices."

30.

Ingest as much as chlorophyll as you can - in the form of salads and greens smoothies, for example! Chlorophyll is the name given to the natural green pigments produced by organisms that carry out photosynthesis. Chlorophyll has one of the best health-promoting properties found on this planet. Chlorophyll stimulates the formation of red blood cells in the bone marrow, rids the organism of environmental toxins such as aflatoxins, slows down cancer cell growth, and has a strong antioxidant effect.

Kale - Chlorella - Spirulina - Parsley - Chinese Cabbage - Wheatgrass - Barley Grass - Spinach - Celery - Broccoli - Lettuce

31.

Eat herbs and wild plants - they boost liver, kidney, and gall bladder function. **Stinging nettle, dandelion, ribwort plantain, ground elder, wild garlic, and coriander** are some of the best-known examples. They support the detoxification process, reduce water retention, are high in nutrients, stimulate your digestion, and are full of valuable, health-promoting secondary metabolites. Plus, they have important anti-inflammatory and antibacterial effects.

32.

Eat sprouts - they have more micronutrients than conventional foods. Choose the sprouts that you like and work them into your meals.

33.

As with milk, **avoid factory farmed meat.** Imagine someone put you in a stable, never let you out, and pumped you full of drugs, antibiotics, and steroids. **Do you think this would be good for your health? Absolutely not! You would be mortally sick.** This is why you should eat organic meat! Factory farmed meat has too many omega-6 and omega-9 fatty acids that increase the risk of inflammation. **Plus, with organic meat being more expensive, you'll automatically eat less.**

Occasional consumption of organic, ethically farmed meat will not do any harm to your health. Moreover, organic meat contains bioavailable amino acids and micronutrients. For those who would refute this on the basis of the China-Study are ignoring the fact that this study is based on research done with animal proteins from factory farmed livestock, which is why this can't be taken as evidence that meat makes people sick in general.

34.

You don't have to go without eggs or fish – as long as they're organic! (smaller fish are less contaminated) Make sure your fish is sustainably farmed.

Fish has valuable omega-3 fatty acids that support brain function, **hinder inflammation,** and stabilize our cells.

35.

Eggs are full of essential nutrients. The assertion that eating eggs increases cholesterol has long been disproved. A single egg contains everything that is needed for a new life (vitamins, minerals, trace elements, amino acids, healthy fats, and more.). It goes without saying that you should opt for organic eggs.

36.

Cook your meals using ghee or coconut oil (refined coconut oil has a neutral flavor). Coconut oil is good for you and has a high smoke point of 350°F.

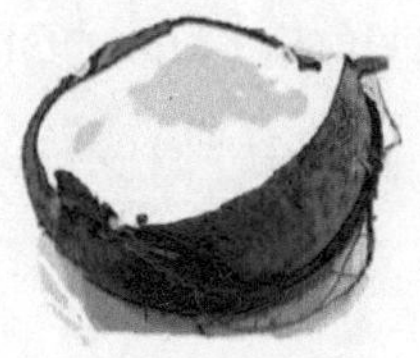

37.

Extra virgin olive oil is also an option but remember: Olive oil is not as heat-resistant as coconut oil at higher temperatures. Olive oil contains the phytochemical oleocanthal. Studies have shown that this plant substance can kill a wide range of cancer cells. People who live on the Mediterranean coast and follow a Mediterranean diet have benefited for centuries from the host of health benefits of high-quality olive oil.

38.

Avoid trans fatty acids. In other words, margarine, frying fat, sunflower oil, safflower oil, soybean oil, and rapeseed oil, whether consumed directly or used in cooking. **Refined products like these mean certain death!** Trans fats are hidden in many processed foods, e.g. in most fast food products, fries, sausage, chips, chocolate, store-bought baked goods, and many more.

Scientific research has shown that trans fats are harmful, increasing LDL cholesterol and lowering HDL cholesterol levels. This can lead to **arteriosclerosis (hardening and narrowing of the arteries) and increases the risk of heart attacks and strokes.** Trans fats damage the brain as a result of severe oxidative stress.

39.

Fat doesn't make you fat!
It's the isolated trans fats
that make you fat, promote
inflammation, and make you sick!
Always choose healthy fats
contained in nuts, seeds,
avocados, eggs, oily fish, black
cumin seed oil, linseed oil, coconut
oil, ghee, or raw milk butter.

40.

When you start making changes
to your diet, you can drink 1 or 2
glasses of water before each
meal to control your hunger.
You will feel full faster, your
bowel function will be stimulated,
and the nutrients can be
absorbed more easily.
You can do that until you've
learnt to control your hunger.

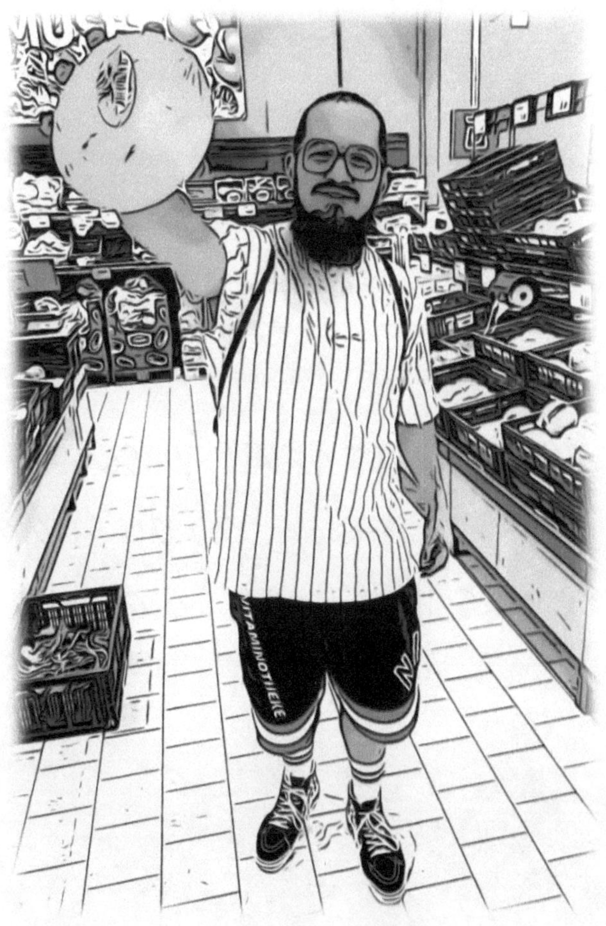

If someone wishes for good health, one must first ask oneself if he is ready to do away with the reasons for his illness. Only then is it possible to help him.

Hippocrates

41.

Store-bought fruit juices make you fat and sick, as do sugary drinks like Coca Cola, etc.

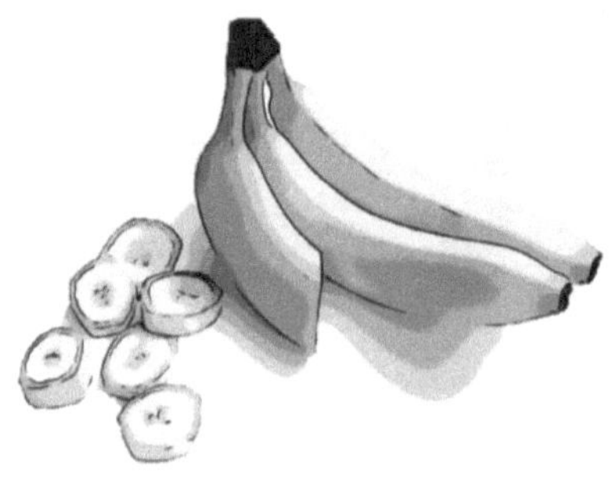

42.

Homemade fruit juices are the better choice because they are fresh and haven't been heated. Store-bought juice might look healthy, but it has still been treated. Always follow the following rule of thumb for smoothies: 80 percent of greens and 20 percent fruit and berries.

43.

Avoid foods with E numbers, artificial coloring, artificial flavoring, and artificial sweeteners.
All of these additives damage your intestines, put your hormones out of balance, and disrupt the regular metabolic processes.

Examples:
Aspartame, Sucralose, Acesulfame K, Glutamate, Tartrazine, Benzoic Acid, Saccharin, or Ammonium Chloride.

44.

If you're wondering **what to cook...**

...buy a cookbook **with vegan, vegetarian, or low-carb recipes, or one with paleo or Mediterranean diet recipes,** or look for suitable recipes online.

45.

Set fixed times for yourself when you consume superfoods. **In the morning right after you get up, during your lunch break, and before you going to bed.** Compared to conventional foods, the nutrient content of superfoods is above average and take your health to the next level:

Avocado - **Pomegranate** - Beetroot - **Papaya** - **Turmeric** - Cocoa - **Algae** - Ginger - **Garlic** - Citrus Fruits - **Berries** - Psyllium Husks - **Cinnamon** - Jerusalem Artichoke - **Spirulina** - Eggs - **Nuts** - Sprouts - **Mushrooms (Maitake and Shiitake)** - Cabbage - **Cruciferae** - Oregano - **Coconut** - Dragon Fruit - **Celery** - Dates - **Olives** - Manuka Honey - **Sidr Honey** - Camel Milk - **Aloe Vera** - Mango - **Bananas** - Pineapple - **Jackfruit** - Mangosteen - **Stevia Leaves** - Broccoli - **Brussels Sprouts**

46.

Know that 80 percent of your immune system is in your gut! It's unimaginable but if your intestines were spread out, it would be several yards long and would cover an area of 300-500 square yards. There are more nerve fibers in the intestines than in the brain! This is why we say: the way to a person's heart is through the stomach! Or: **"This problem leaves me with an awful feeling in the pit of my stomach!"** The enteric nerve system found inside the intestines is often referred to as the body's second brain, the gut-brain axis.

You have more gut bacteria in your body than cells, so make sure to nourish your intestines with lactic acid bacteria (probiotics/prebiotics) and plenty of fiber (vegetables, psyllium husks, flaxseed meal, sauerkraut, Jerusalem artichoke, inulin). These will improve your gut health and keep your gut fit. **Your gut bacteria produce important vitamins** and make sure that other important nutrients are absorbed.

Your brain produces 50 percent of the "feel-good hormone" dopamine while the remaining 50 percent is produced by the intestines. Many people don't know that only 5 percent of the happy hormone serotonin is produced by the brain, with the remaining 95 percent being produced by the intestine. It is important to know that your mood depends primarily on your gut health.

 Soak nuts, seeds, pseudograins, and grains in water for several hours. This neutralizes adverse properties, reduces the concentration of antinutrients, and makes them easier to digest. Don't forget to consume as much fermented food as possible. Fermentation is one of the most important processes used in ancient times to stop food from spoiling and to bring about health benefits. You can ferment food yourself or buy fermented products in the store.

What does "fermentation" mean?

Fermentation is a process where food is placed in salt water, and put in a covered container to create an environment in which lactic acid can grow, and where the growth of harmful bacteria is prevented. Fermentation requires microorganisms such as bacteria and fungi. Microorganisms convert large molecules into small ones, extracting energy from them. In a sense, fermentation is something like a digestive process where microorganisms break down organic molecules to draw energy from them.

What do fermented foods contain?

Fermented foods contain enzymes and active lactic acid bacteria that create a balanced environment in the intestines, boosting and regulating your immune system. Besides enzymes and lactic acid bacteria, fermented foods also contain various vitamins and phytochemicals that have an antioxidative effect and boost the immune system. They are greatly beneficial to many areas of the body, counteracting diseases such as cancer, diabetes, and cardiovascular diseases. Fermented foods also prevent cravings, as they contain fewer harmful microorganisms.

47.

Don't be too hard on yourself! Treat yourself once a week to something you fancy, even if it isn't the healthiest of choices! Eating something unhealthy once a week when you're in company won't kill you: **"The dose makes the poison."**

48.

Respect doctors and their work and take their advice seriously. But remember that doctors are only human beings who can make mistakes or who are compelled to make mistakes, for whatever reason. Never forget to get a second opinion! You have to take responsibility for your own health. Nobody else can take on that responsibility – regardless of who. Don't let anybody scare you. Fear weakens your immune system immensely and manipulates your intuition and individual capacity to make decisions.

Use your brain and get on top of your health
or your illness for that matter.
Own it! That way you won't have to pass
the responsibility on to anyone else.
Alternatively, you should strive to find the
right doctors or therapists – ones that
have a keen **sense of responsibility** and are
passionate about helping people.

Immanuel Kant said:
"Dare to know! Have the courage to use your
own intelligence!"

49.

Paracelsus

Nobody has to stop eating meat!
Nobody has to start eating meat!
Carbohydrates are neither bad nor good.
**What makes them good or bad is how
we look at them.** Don't follow every
nutritional "pseudoscience" religiously.
The next "diet fad" will come along the
next day and change everything again.
No one should be tied down to any food
or diet ideology.
Never forget: **"The dose of everything
you put in your mouth makes the
poison!"**

50.

Avoid stress!

"The problem is not the problem; but the problem is your attitude about the problem!"
(It's about how you look at things and handle them.)
- Captain Jack Sparrow

Mindset is everything!

Why should I avoid stress caused by **an unhealthy diet** and stress caused by **an unstable state of mind?**

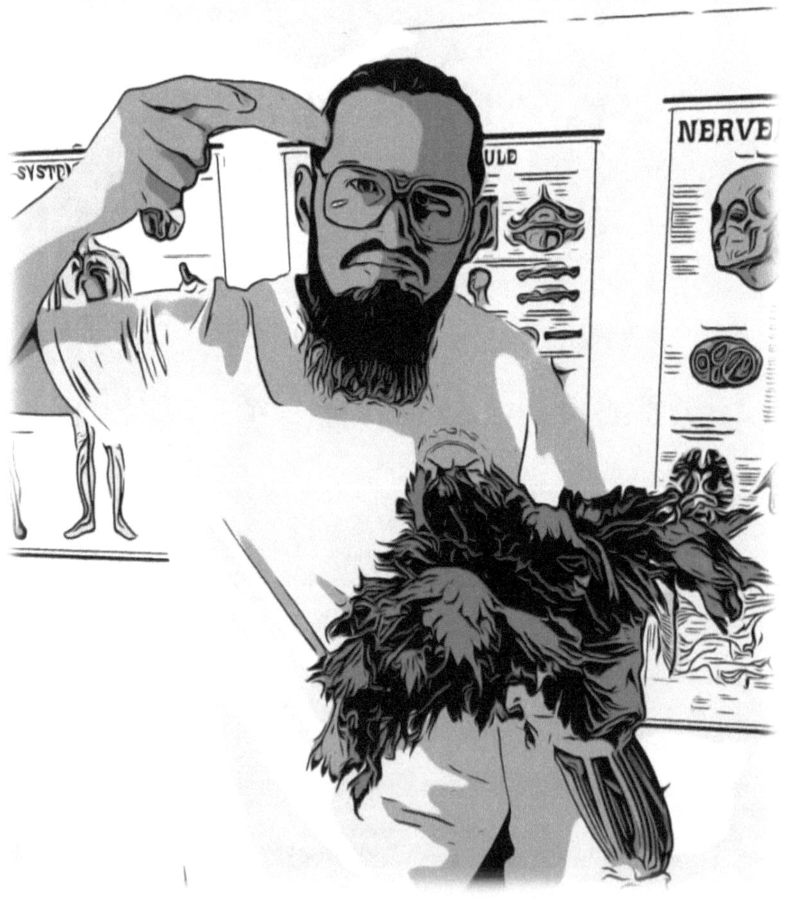

Now that you've become familiar with the principles of nutrition, let's take a look at another important cornerstone of your health: Your mind!

The mind is regarded separately from the body (society is to blame for this). This, however, is a common misconception that is also denied by western medicine.

In other words, we have been misled by the assumption that our mind has no influence on our body and therefore no influence on our health. But what about what is known as clinical psychoneuroimmunology, a science that deals with the interaction between the mind and the immune system and looks at the neurological factors that contribute to this interaction. Traumas are a perfect example of this interaction. Trauma can be both physiological and psychological.

A psychological trauma is a psychological wound that arises as a result of an imbalance between a forbidding situation and your mental capacity to cope with this situation. This situation is accompanied by a feeling of helplessness and vulnerability.

If we look at our everyday lives, we will begin to see a pattern emerge. A pattern of subconscious and unbroken routines and habits. If this pattern is suddenly interrupted - say by a traumatic experience - our system is overwhelmed and can't deal with the potential "threat".

Death is a typical example of trauma. The unexpected death of a loved one interrupts our usual pattern and we feel helpless, not knowing how to react to make things better. The consequence: We succumb to our emotions.

It should be said at this point that mourning is absolutely advisable. That said, some people are less resilient than others, meaning their mental state will not allow them to return to day-to-day challenges after an appropriate period of mourning.

And if we get stuck in our emotions, our immune system will be hugely affected. The reason for this is that cell function depends on the information the cells receive. If our mind believes that we are in a threatening situation, it sends a signal to our cells, telling them that the environment isn't helping us at the moment. A sudden death, which interrupts the established pattern, is seen as such a threat. This threat then triggers stress!

The system responsible for this biochemical mechanism is called the **hypothalamus-pituitary-adrenal axis or the HPA axis. The hypothalamus is the part of the brain that interprets perceptual function.** If the hypothalamus gauges a situation as stressful, it passes it on to the pituitary gland, which in turn sends the signal to the adrenal gland, stimulating it to produce stress hormones.

The adrenal gland is the very organ which then initiates the fight-or-flight response. **In other words, these stress hormones put us in a physical state where we are prepared either to fight or to flee. We are mentally alert and quick to find solutions.**

In this state, our remaining energy resources and our blood are taken away from our organs and pumped into our muscles. If our organs are not supplied with blood and the necessary energy, our body will not be willing to grow, heal or maintain health.

The stress hormones cause our cells to close! Our cells do this to protect themselves from the imminent threat – and remain closed until the perceived risk has gone. What this means, however, is that the individual cells no longer work properly.

Our intestine is home to our immune system. Stress and the reluctance of the cells prevents the intestine from doing its job, creating a breeding ground for germs, bacteria, and viruses that live in our intestines, kept in check by our immune system. **When we experience stress, however, our immune system shuts down. Stress over longer periods of time is therefore not only harmful but might lead to the collapse of the entire organism.**

But to come back to our example once again: When a loved one dies our everyday routine is disrupted so severely that we are overwhelmed by the situation. This results in stress which, in turn, puts us into survival mode. We can do without everything, even a functioning organism and immune system - as long as we can survive.

When our life is at stake, we have the choice between fighting the current situation to find our way back into everyday life or taking flight, rejecting the reality, denying what we have lost and running away. **If we choose the latter option, we create the perfect breeding ground for germs, bacteria, and viruses.**

Since we can't run away from the things that catch up with us time and again, harmless acute stress turns into permanent chronic stress. If we are unable to rid ourselves of the trauma, chronic stress will accompany us throughout our lives. This chronic stress is one of the main causes of physical and mental sickness.

Having created the ideal conditions, we 'breed' diseases which we then detect too late. **Cancer** is one of the most well-known diseases commonly diagnosed too late.

Of course, not everybody is, and you may well not be, a victim of such trauma, but let me conclude by saying one thing: The example mentioned here may sound extreme; trauma does not always have to result from such an extreme experience or situation.

Basically, almost anything can cause stress. We are living in an era in which chronic stress has become a widespread disease. Constantly failing to live up the ever-increasing demands imposed by society, our own lives have become a struggle we feel we can no longer manage. **This is due to the stimuli we get from the environment every day. Just think – today we are exposed to as many environmental stimuli in one day as people centuries ago were exposed to throughout their entire lives.** We are so inundated with stimuli that we become overwhelmed and our mind is no longer able to cope with this hectic world. And, as mentioned earlier, such overwhelming situations result in stress. We experience these symptoms when we are already stressed by everyday life or if we worry too much. Whether this happens or not essentially comes down to us, but we must engage our minds and our intellect. For the mind and intellect are the sources of our stress, our fears, and our worries. Once we have those under control and have understood the connections, our health will be in our own hands.

I hope that I have succeeded in showing you that we have to see our health, or rather ourselves, as a whole. Sticking to these nutritional principles will give you a solid foundation, but it can only be fully successful if we bring our minds into the equation, too. Disregarding the mind shows how little we understand about health and the human body.

Consider this book an opportunity to rethink and take stock of your current situation. You might be stressed by something, maybe by a task you don't feel up to at the moment. The first thing that can help reduce these stress factors is Emotional Intelligence. This topic would go beyond the scope of this book, but it would definitely help you to deal with the factors mentioned.
Always remember:

"We cannot solve our problems with the same thinking we used to create them." - Albert Einstein.

Andreas Simons
Author of the chapter "Avoid stress!"
Responsible for the sections on "Psychokinesiology"
and "Psychoneuroimmunology" (PNI) at "Vitaminotheke" in Germany.
Instagram: _Andreassimons

Proteins

Proteins are instrumental in the human body. Proteins have an energy density of 4 kcal/g and are the vital building blocks of cell production and regeneration. Each protein consists of different amino acids, which can be found in every enzyme in the body, making them essential for our metabolism. In most conventional diets, protein is neglected, despite the central role it plays in the body's detoxification or repair processes.

Plant proteins	Animal proteins
Quinoa	Organic eggs
Spirulina	Fish (especially salmon, cod, mahi-mahi, trout; always go for quality)
Chlorella	
Pulses	Beef (except conventional supermarket quality)
Nuts	
Soy	Lamb (lean)
Clean, natural protein shakes	Poultry (organic)
Lupine	Seafood (good quality)
	Veal
	Dairy products (organic raw milk only)

Carbohydrates

Carbohydrates or "carbs," which supply our body with energy, come in the form of short- and long-chain carbohydrates, from simple sugars to sweet potatoes or rice. Carbohydrates also have an energy density of 4 kcal/gr and are metabolized differently. Short-chain carbohydrates have a higher insulin response because the blood sugar level increases faster than with long-chain carbohydrates. Eating mainly short-chain carbohydrates means that the blood sugar level will be subject to heavy fluctuations, leading to hunger attacks. A healthy diet should keep your blood sugar at a constant level. Increased fiber consumption and long-chain carbs can help with this.

Long-chain carbohydrates
Sweet potato
Quinoa
Brown rice
Pumpkin
Amaranth
Millet
Basmati rice
Gluten-free grain
Manioc
Black rice
Yams
Vegetables

Fats

Fat doesn't make you "fat"!

Fat is a very important component in the production of our hormones. "Saturated fat," despite its bad reputation, is essential for the production of our sex hormones. if you tend to use a lot of butter and lard, try replacing them with coconut oil or high-quality butter, for example. Our body needs fats to build and preserve cells, and fats are an important source of energy for the body. Fats have an energy density of 9 kcal/g. Besides saturated fatty acids, there are also monounsaturated fatty acids (such as olive oil and nuts, which should never be heated) and polyunsaturated fatty acids (omega-3 and omega-6).

Healthy fats	
Hemp seeds	Olive oil
Pumpkin seeds	Omega-3 fatty acids
Sesame	Nut oils
Sunflower seeds	Linseed oil
Ghee	Coconut oil
Hemp oil	Nuts and nut butter
Egg yolk	Egg yolk
Avocados	Raw milk butter

Micronutrients are absolutely indispensable for metabolism.
In other words: They are the software for our body.
Without them, diseases and imbalances can occur in the body.
What would our laptops and smartphones be without software? They wouldn't work! Just like your body can't work without micronutrients. There are different types of micronutrients:

- Vitamins
- Minerals
- Trace elements
- Phytochemicals
- Amino acids
- Enzymes

<u>Today's major causes of micronutrient deficiency:</u>

1. <u>Monoculture foods</u>, where depleted soils are lacking in micronutrients.

2. <u>Hybrid and genetically modified foods</u>, i.e. foods cultivated to have a certain appearance, a specific taste or to produce higher yields.

3. <u>Pesticides</u>, which disrupt the metabolic processes in food, meaning micronutrients can't be absorbed from the soil.

4. <u>Harvesting too early or at the wrong time</u>. All foods that are harvested too early or at the wrong time have major deficiencies in their micronutrient balance.

5. <u>Medication:</u> Change the gastric environment, impeding the absorption of nutrients. Plus, in order to get to where they are needed, drugs manipulate your metabolism to such an extent that severe nutrient loss occurs in the cells.

Thanks to all these factors, lettuce and cucumber from the supermarket have as many micronutrients as a Kleenex!

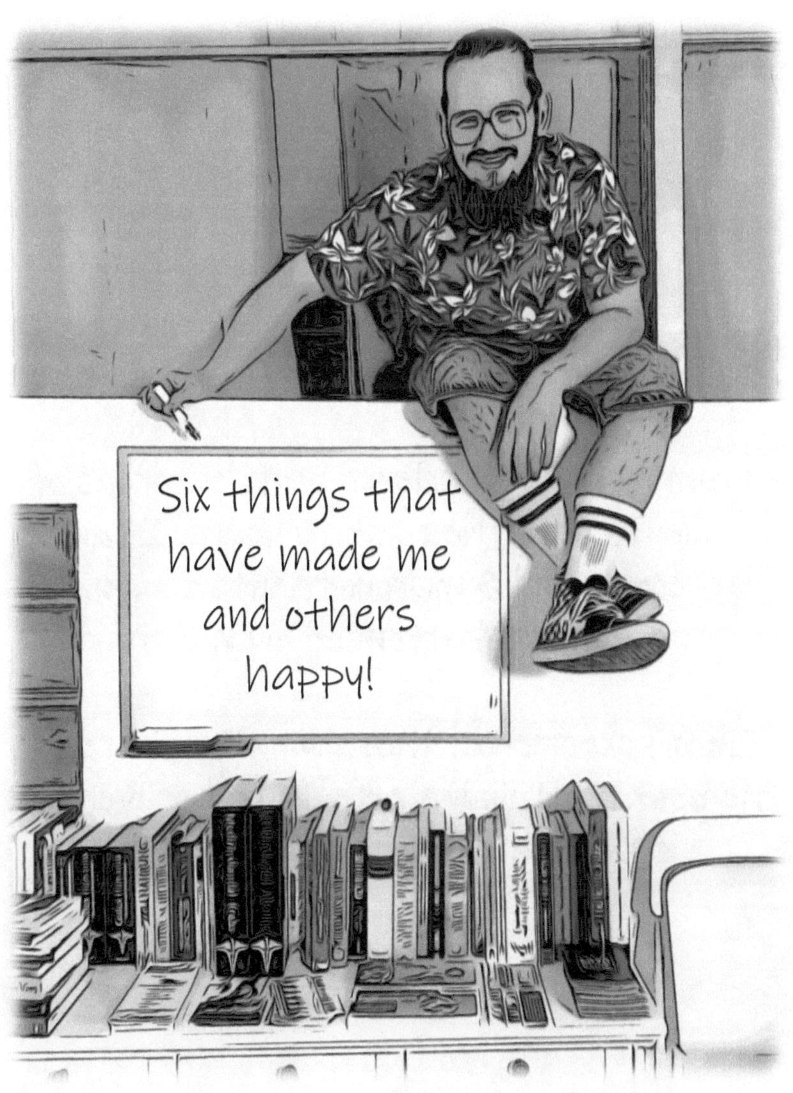
Six things that have made me and others happy!

A matter of the heart for me!

From my own experience with hundreds of clients over the past 10 years, I can recommend 6 micronutrients to you. From the bottom of my heart!

In my experience, these 6 nutrients reap the best revitalizing effects and deliver the best results over the long term.

Linus Pauling

To quote the laureate of the Nobel Prize for Chemistry and one of the greatest, best known orthomolecular scientists of all time (1901 - 1994):

I believe that, by taking some simple and inexpensive measures, you can lead a long and healthy life. The one crucial recommendation I can make is that you add to the vitamins that you get from your food by taking the necessary quantities of supplements every day.

Vitamin D

Vitamin D is a fat-soluble vitamin which is often referred to as the "sunshine hormone". Vitamin D is not an ordinary vitamin, but rather a hormone and is not absorbed primarily through food. In fact, vitamin D is formed under the skin after exposure to UVB radiation from the sun. Vitamin D is responsible, for example, for the absorption of calcium in the body, i.e., it ensures that the calcium present in the intestine can be absorbed at all. You could say that calcium is ineffective without vitamin D. Every cell in our body has a receptor for vitamin D, indicating that every cell NEEDS vitamin D.

Hormonal Effects

Strictly speaking, vitamin D is not a vitamin. In fact, after metabolism the active form of vitamin D is a hormone. As mentioned before, it is not absorbed primarily through food, but through the skin, with the help of UVB rays from the sun. Muscle contraction, cold, and bioavailable magnesium are co-factors in the activation of vitamin D.

Vitamin D
- activates more than 2000 genes
- ensures healthy bone metabolism
- influences cell differentiation
- helps stabilize our mood
- activates the immune system
- helps regulate hormonal balance
- helps to maintain muscle function
- has an anti-inflammatory effect
- helps regulate the nervous system
- helps stabilize the autonomic nervous system
- helps maintain mental health and cognition
- supports bone, joint, and tendon health

What level of vitamin D should we have?

Toxic effect	over 300 ng/ml
Risk of too high or increased calcium level	over 150 ng/ml
Recommended maximum level in the blood	100 ng/ml
Regular sunbathing	50-90 ng/ml
Ideal level (minimal risk of disease)	50-90 ng/ml
Good level (low risk of disease)	over 40 ng/ml
Reasonable level (good calcium absorption)	over 30 ng/ml
Deficiency (risk of osteoporosis in old age)	under 30 ng/ml
Severe deficiency (high risk of osteoporosis, disorder of the autonomic nervous system)	under 20 ng/ml
Extreme deficiency (osteomalacia, rickets)	under 12 ng/ml

Do we get enough vitamin D?

Our primary source of vitamin D is UVB rays. Some 80-90 percent of our vitamin D needs comes from exposure to UVB, with as little as 5-20 percent coming from food. This means that food is not a noteworthy factor for good or optimal vitamin D intake! But what about UVB radiation? Cities located at 51 degrees latitude, for example, receive too little UVB radiation, even in summer. This is the reason for severe vitamin D deficiency (24 ng/ml) in many people, to say nothing of the months from October to March, where we don't receive any vitamin D at all (the average level in winter is 8 ng/ml!). The annual average vitamin D level in Germany, for example, is about 16 ng/ml! People who live at latitudes where they get frequent sun exposure avoid the sun and have poor vitamin D levels. It is therefore very important to check the vitamin D level in your blood if you have health problems. This will help you rule out any possible harm caused by vitamin D deficiency and take countermeasures. The daily dosage for adults is 10,000 IU -20,000 IU.
Cofactors: 200 micrograms of vitamin K2 taken in combination with 200 - 300 milligrams of magnesium every morning and evening.

Symptoms of vitamin D deficiency

<u>Acute symptoms of vitamin D deficiency</u>
- Muscle pain and muscle weakness
- Chronic listlessness and exhaustion
- Functional neurological disorder, resulting in sleep disorders, constant fatigue, and lethargy
- Circulation problems, feeling cold (especially your hands and feet)
- Osteoporosis and osteomalacia (softening and weakening of the bones)

The role of vitamin D in disease prevention:

- Autoimmune diseases
- Diabetes
- Cardiovascular diseases
- High blood pressure
- Articular rheumatism
- Muscle weakness
- Autoimmune diseases
- Rheumatoid arthritis
- Neurological diseases
- Chronic inflammation
- Mental illness
- Osteoporosis
- Common cold
- PMS
- Bone diseases
- Back and bone pain
- Cancer

Vitamin K2

Vitamin K2 is a fat-soluble vitamin which is synthesized by gut bacteria or ingested through food.

Function:

Vitamin K2 prevents soft-tissue calcification, supports bone regeneration and mineralization, and transports calcium to its intended place (bones, muscles, teeth, brain, etc.). Vitamin K2 contains the transport molecule that ensures that calcium ingested through food is introduced into the bones and retained there (Vitamin D plays a central role in the metabolism of calcium). It prevents hypercalcemia and makes sure that the calcium is incorporated where it belongs.

Vitamin K2 and oral health

By the way, an acute K2 deficiency in children can often lead to tooth decay. Interestingly, animals and "uncivilized" peoples have completely healthy teeth, i.e., no tooth decay or other dental problems - and they don't even brush their teeth! The reason why people have bad teeth is that the jawbone is too narrow, meaning that too little calcium has been stored during childhood. In parts of the world where people get enough vitamin K2, crooked teeth and bones are neither common nor normal.

where can this vitamin be found?
Vitamin K2 can only be found in animal fats such as cheese,
meat, milk, butter, and egg yolks - as long as the animals
have grazed on green grass.
But even then, it is hard to tell whether this is enough to
ensure you cover your basic vitamin K requirements.

How do we absorb it?
It is unclear whether the amount of K2 absorbed into the
blood from the gut is sufficient. Your body can only partly
convert vitamin K1 absorbed through food into vitamin K2,
which is important for our health. In addition, many
people's gut flora is disrupted by antibiotics, an unhealthy
diet, increasingly sterile environments, and poor hygiene.
Daily vitamin K2 requirement for adults: 200 micrograms.

Vitamin C

Vitamin C, also known as ascorbic acid, is a water-soluble antioxidant which we absorb through our food (especially fruit and vegetables).

Vitamin C helps our:

immune system – cardiovascular system - protect the metabolism from free radicals - hormone production – fat metabolism - production of neurotransmitters - reduction of inflammatory mediators - regulation of gene expression

What do we need vitamin C for?

Vitamin C is involved in 15,000 metabolic processes - from hormone production to fat metabolism, nothing works without vitamin C. This vitamin is also essential for the production of neurotransmitters.

Vitamin C is particularly abundant in the liver, muscles, and the brain. It is also very important for iron absorption in the body and helps enable its mobilization from storage.

Vitamin C is the body's most important nutrient after water and oxygen. Recommendation for adults: A total of 1-2 grams taken throughout the day - sodium ascorbate, calcium ascorbate, ascorbyl palmitate, camu camu, acerola cherry, sweet pepper, or citrus fruits.

Vitamin C reduces the risk of cardiovascular diseases

Vitamin C captures free radicals and protects absorbed lipids from oxidation. It can also take over free radicals from other antioxidants (e.g. vitamin E) in order to prepare them for use again.

Fewer free radicals mean fewer inflammatory mediators, which is one of the main causes of cardiovascular diseases. Vitamin C can help repair damage to the artery walls, allowing them to expand under higher pressure and preventing dangerous micro-tears in the arteries. Vitamin C helps lower blood pressure, reducing the risk of strokes and arteriosclerosis.

Circulation and the central nervous system

By combatting free radicals, vitamin C provides long-term protection for the 100 billion neurons in the central nervous system, reducing the risk of a stroke and thus the risk of brain damage.

Vitamin C and cancer

The US National Cancer Research Institute evaluated 47 clinical studies on the effects of vitamin C: 34 studies showed a high vitamin C content in the blood to decrease the risk of cancer by 50 percent.

Zinc

The human body contains about 1.5 - 2.5 grams of zinc. The body can't produce this trace element itself, which is why it has to be supplied regularly through food. Zinc regulates the build-up and break-down of proteins, fats, and carbohydrates.

It is important for:

cell proliferation - cell protection - immune system - skin, hair & nails – the release of neurotransmitters - wound healing – acid-base balance regulation - formation and storage of insulin.

Immune system

Zinc plays an important role in immune cell proliferation and has an anti-inflammatory effect. At the same time, it is an antioxidant, which combats free radicals.

Skin, hair & nails

Zinc is essential for the formation of healthy skin cells and the production of collagen, which is one of the most important building blocks for the skin. Zinc is also instrumental in the production of keratin. It is this protein molecule that makes your hair and nails firm.

Recommendation for adults: 25 milligrams daily (not on an empty stomach)

Natural messenger substances

Zinc is necessary for the formation of messenger substances such as neurotransmitters and hormones such as the well-known testosterone. This trace element is also crucial for the development of the male sex organs and sperm production. Like men, women need zinc to produce sex hormones and guarantee fertility.

The benefits of citrate

- Better zinc absorption
- Reduced acid load (e.g. of the kidney cells), which protects the kidneys
- Higher urine pH value
- Reduced risk of kidney stones
- Helps dissolve kidney stones

Magnesium

Magnesium is one of the ten most common elements in the Earth's crust. An abundance of magnesium can also be found in chlorophyll. Approx. 400 enzymes are dependent on magnesium, which means that magnesium has a direct and indirect influence on metabolic processes.

The importance of magnesium:

essential for bones - skeletal muscle - teeth - cells - metabolism - nervous system - blood pressure stabilization - vitamin D activation – helps stimulate gut activity – stabilizes sugar metabolism

Can we get enough magnesium from our food?

An average person needs about 400-500 mg of magnesium a day. As little as 200 mg, however, is obtained from fruits and vegetables. One of the main reasons for this widespread deficiency is the fact that there is hardly any magnesium left in the depleted soils. Plus, if we consume products like milk, cheese, or yogurt, which are high in calcium, our body needs even more magnesium to maintain the optimum balance between calcium and magnesium. Furthermore, magnesium is one of the minerals that is quickly utilized in the cells. Stress and intense physical exertion speed up metabolism, and the magnesium is excreted from your body. For optimum magnesium levels in the body, it is important to avoid calcium overload so that the magnesium in the cells can increase.

Magnesium supplements

Supplements such as magnesium citrate, magnesium bisglycinate, or magnesium malate are easily soluble and can be absorbed easily by the body.

The unique effects of magnesium citrate:
- Better magnesium absorption
- Reduced acid load (e.g. of the kidney cells), which protects the kidneys
- Higher urine pH value
- Reduced risk of kidney stones
- Helps dissolve kidney stones

The unique effects of magnesium bisglycinate:
- Improved magnesium absorption
- Highly absorbable amino acid compound (glycine)
- Calming and relaxing effect on the central nerve system, because magnesium binds to the receptors in the glycine compound
- Glycine improves the quality of your sleep, meaning you will feel more rested when you wake

The unique effects of magnesium malate:
- Better magnesium absorption
- Improved enzyme activity, resulting in improved cellular energy production; the mitochondrial energy supply is increased.

Intake

Magnesium intake should be spread over the day:
First part of the dose: in the morning after getting up.
Last part of the dose: one or two hours before bedtime.
When you eat food containing calcium, it is important to take extra magnesium to restore the ratio between calcium and magnesium.

Transdermal absorption

The external use of magnesium salts is a long-standing tradition, especially for skin disorders or joint complaints. Magnesium baths (full or foot baths) can be carried out at home with magnesium chloride. Make sure that the magnesium concentration is high, and always soak for at least half an hour. It is also possible to mix magnesium chloride with oil, which creates an oil-like consistency that can then be applied to the skin.

Advantages of transdermal (lit. "on the skin") absorption compared to oral intake:

- Fast and direct absorption
- Improved healing and activated immune response against wounds and eczema.

Omega-3 fatty acids

Omega-3 fatty acids belong to the group of unsaturated
fatty acids. These essential nutrients can't be synthesized
(produced) by the body, meaning they must be ingested
through food.

Tasks/important for:

cell membrane stabilization - brain tissue growth and
function - cell communication - formation of serotonin - has a
positive effect on the mind/mood - alleviates joint pain and
arthritis symptoms - reduces inflammation – boosts the
effect of vitamins E, D, K and A.

Omega-3 fatty acids and our brain

Approximately 60 percent of our brain tissue consists of
fats, 25 percent of which is DHA (Docosahexaenoic acid).
Omega-3 fatty acids are important for communication
between cells, which is why memory loss is linked to Omega-
3 deficiency. Omega-3 fats have been found to help reverse
degenerative states. One study showed a daily intake of
900 mg DHA over a period of 24 weeks to bring about
significant improvements in brain function, levels of
inflammation, and mental health when compared to the
control group in the study.

Omega-3 fatty acids and neck or back pain

Researchers at a US university discovered that 60 percent of patients with neck and back pain no longer had to take painkillers after replacing ibuprofen with 1.2 grams of omega-3 fish oil a day. What must be noted, however, is that the fatty acids cease to have any effect the minute you fry fish. Frying produces trans fats and oxidized aldehydes which damage the heart and brain.

Omega-3 fatty acids and depression

Docosahexaenoic acid (DHA) facilitates the release of serotonin and strengthens the neural membrane – hence its antidepressant effect. Recent studies have shown that omega-3 deficiency in the blood can lead to mental and emotional problems such as depression, anxiety disorders, and schizophrenia.

Omega-3 fatty acids and joint pain
Combining fish oil with other natural substances can
alleviate joint pain.

These natural substances are:
- Type II collagen
- Glucosamine
- Chondroitin
- Cissus Quadrangularis
- MSM (organic sulfur)
- To alleviate arthritis symptoms and joint pain in adults,
  the ideal dosage is about 3 grams of fish oil per day. If
  taken for treatment purposes, however, this dosage,
  cannot be achieved solely by eating fish.

Taking omega-3 fatty acids is recommended for health problems such as:
Alzheimer's disease - asthma - arthrosis - ADHD - high
blood pressure - depression - dementia - cardiovascular
diseases - obesity - rheumatoid arthritis - cancer - multiple
sclerosis - osteoporosis – neurological and inflammatory
diseases (where they are found to be particularly beneficial).

It is important to make sure that the omega-3 fatty
acids you ingest are of high quality meaning low heavy
metal contamination. Another alternative: Krill oil

You might have to
do without that
extra pair of
sneakers, but in
return you'll be in
the best of health."

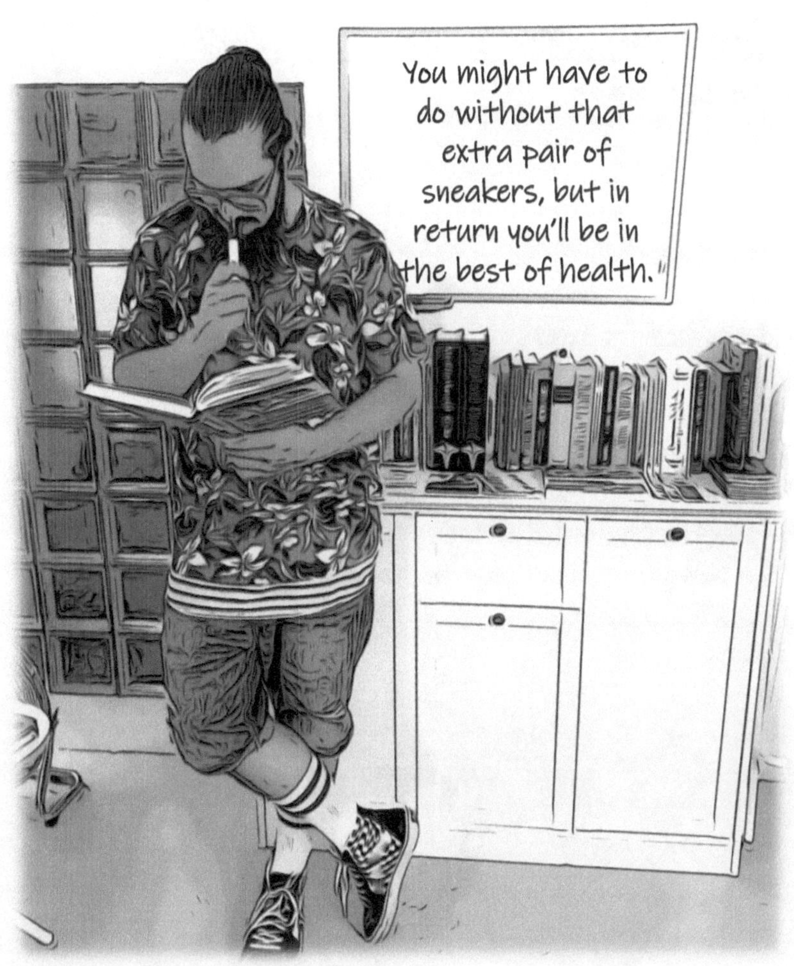

130

<u>Detox & anti-aging & disease prevention</u>
Chlorella algae
The word 'chlorella' derives from Latin and means something along the lines of "small, young green". Chlorella is a particular type of algae that grows in freshwater and has a single cell nucleus (unlike spirulina and AFA algae). This type of algae is exceptionally rich in nutrients and help rid the body of toxins.

It is the adaptability of this complex unicellular organism that makes it so interesting to scientists and has allowed it to survive for well over two million years. Algae is one of the best researched organisms. Chlorella algae is available as a powder or in supplement form.

Tasks:
detoxifies - strengthens the immune system - counteracts iron deficiency - stimulates hematopoietic response - has anti-inflammatory effects - improves digestion - anti-carcinogenic - supports liver function - increases protein supply - improves gut activity through high fiber content - removes heavy metals from the body.

Vitamins contained in chlorella:

- Vitamin B1
- Vitamin B2
- Vitamin B5
- Vitamin B6
- Biotin
- Vitamin B12
- Vitamin C
- Vitamin D
- Vitamin E

Minerals and trace elements:

- Calcium
- Magnesium
- Potassium
- Manganese
- Iodine
- Phosphorous
- Iron
- Zinc
- Copper

Essential fatty acids

Chlorella algae contain 30 different fatty acids, meaning about one third of all types of fatty acids (saturated, unsaturated, and polyunsaturated fatty acids).

Binders for toxins and contaminants

Thanks to the cell structure of Chlorella algae, they help the body rid itself of contaminants (heavy metals and other toxins) by binding them and excreting them through your stool.

Chlorophyll

Chlorophyll can also be called the "green in the leaf" of a plant. Its chemical structure is similar to that of hemoglobin (red blood pigment) in the human body. This is why chlorophyll is the best nutrient for our blood. To date, no other plant has been found to contain as much chlorophyll as Chlorella algae.

Protection for the liver

Chlorophyll protects the liver cells from toxins (regardless of whether they are dental toxins, fungal infections, environmental toxins, or food contaminated with pesticides).

What effect does chlorophyll in Chlorella algae have?
- Better protection and increased regenerative capacity for every cell in the body, increasing cell lifespan and noticeably slowing down the aging process.
- Improves circulation and boosts the digestive system
- Restores the acid base balance (alkaline)
- Antioxidant effect (protection against free radicals), preventing inflammatory reactions and counteracting cell degeneration (incl. in the gut)
- Carcinogenic toxins are bound, forming an insoluble "mixture" that is excreted via the intestine.

Additional health benefits for your body
- Increased cellular respiration (increased oxygen content in the blood)
- Activates metabolism
- Protection of the cell walls
- Balances the release of digestive juices
- Support for all healing processes
- Serenity and inner peace

Please note:

This dietary supplement is not suitable for everyone. Women who are pregnant or nursing, in particular, should not take additional chlorella! It is not recommended for children or teenagers either!
As long as you do not exceed the recommended dose, adults (unless pregnant) do not have to worry about any side effects.

N.B.:

Here is an important note on the cultivation of Chlorella algae. Under no circumstances should products be used which grow in areas of high concern and contamination! It is not unusual for products from China to be contaminated with heavy metals, industrial toxins, pesticides, and cadmium. Such products are very bad to your health and very toxic to the organism. They can also cause nerve or brain damage, cancer, or other diseases.

MSM organic sulfur

This sulfur compound, methylsulfonylmethane (MSM sulfur), is not a very well-known nutrient - and yet, it is one of the most important minerals of all. MSM can be found in many animal or plant organisms. Sulfur makes up 0.2 percent of the body and is therefore more abundant than, for example, the trace element iron or the vital mineral magnesium.

It is important for:

healthy stomach mucosa (to stop parasites from settling) - positive effect on acidic stomach - metabolism stimulation – detoxification in the body - supports the immune system - cell wall formation - tissue - joints - muscles - natural painkiller - anti-inflammatory

The effects of MSM sulfur

The body uses MSM sulfur to produce various enzymes, amino acids, and hormones.

Detoxification, protein metabolism, and the build-up of connective tissue are not possible without MSM sulfur!

In combination with oxygen, other vitamins (e.g. vitamin C), and minerals, MSM sulfur has a stronger and more targeted effect, so using this product will not have a huge effect.

MSM sulfur is used for the following complaints:
allergies - arthrosis and arthritis - chronic muscle and joint
pain - migraine – fungal infections and parasite infestation -
heartburn - constipation - diabetes - rheumatism - muscle
soreness and muscle pain in general - detoxification -
glutathione synthesis

Symptoms of deficiency
Being somewhat indeterminable, individual symptoms cannot
be easily attributed to a lack of MSM.

Possible symptoms of MSM deficiency:
liver problems – circulation problems - depression and feeling
down - joint problems - anxiety - pale skin - brittle
fingernails - weak connective tissue - dry, dull hair - allergies

Dosage and intake

According to the American Food and Drug Administration (FDA), a maximum daily dosage of 4 grams of MSM sulfur is a harmless dietary supplement. Patients suffering from arthrosis or other types of inflammation can initially take 2-3 grams a day. If you have severe pain, 4 grams a day may be taken temporarily; this dosage may even be increased to 10 grams a day.

Important:

This dietary supplement is not suitable for everyone. Pregnant women or nursing mothers, in particular, should not take MSM sulfur! It isn't recommended for children and teenagers either!
As long as you do not exceed the recommended dose, adults (unless pregnant) do not have to worry about any side effects.

Transdermal application of MSM sulfur

It is recommended to use MSM ointment to treat acne, redness, or severe itching. Apply the ointment on the affected areas 2 to 3 times a day. The ointment can also be used for joint and muscle pains.

OPC grape seed extract (GSE)

OPC (oligomeric proanthocyanidin), also known as vitamin P, is a phytochemical or secondary metabolite that was discovered in 1948. It is considered to be the best vascular protection and one of the strongest antioxidants. OPC is 100% bioavailable and protects the cells from free radicals. Grape seed extract is 50 times more antioxidative than vitamin E, i.e., 50 times more effective than vitamin E in protecting cells from free radicals. In addition, it is 20 times more effective than vitamin C - this is reason enough to learn more about this secondary metabolite. Anyone can take OPC, whether old or young. It is also safe for pregnant women (although they should ensure that the OPC has come from grapes and not pine bark). If taken during pregnancy, OPC can boost the unborn child's immune systems and improve circulation in the placenta.

Positive effect on:

blood circulation - detoxification of the body - resistance of blood vessels stroke prevention) - cardiovascular system - blood lipids - blood sugar balance - eyes - allergies - skin (acne, neurodermatitis, dry skin) - elasticity of toenails and fingernails - wounds and bone injuries - cancer - degenerative aging processes (Alzheimer's disease, dementia, memory loss, Parkinson's disease) - respiratory tract - mood (depression, learning and concentration difficulties, etc.) - immune system - kidney - osteoporosis - liver

Where can OPC be found?
- Grape seeds
- Green tea
- Strawberries
- Blueberries
- Red grapes
- Apples
- Pine bark of the maritime pine
- Red peanut skins

Dosage and intake
The daily dosage of OPC is 250-300 mg (in capsule form) or ½ teaspoon of powder.

The recommendation is approximately 3 mg per kg of body weight, maximum 5 mg.

OPC should be taken approx. 30 minutes after breakfast or lunch.

Tip: Always take OPC in combination with vitamin C! This can boost the effect of vitamin C considerably – by as much as ten times!

Those who need more OPC:
Smokers who ingest large amounts of toxins or patients with cancer have an increased need for this nutrient. I recommend consulting a physician about your individual requirements. At this point I would like to draw your attention to the fact that anyone taking more than 300 mg daily should be monitored by a physician. The desired effects of OPC usually manifest after 4 - 8 weeks, depending on the person's diet and health.

OPC and cancer
Studies published since 1994 show that OPC can positively impact intestinal and breast cancer. Grape seed extract can prevent the growth of various types of cancer, such as stomach, intestinal, breast, and prostate cancer. Studies carried out by the University of Colorado Cancer Center and the Skaggs School of Pharmaceutical Sciences found that OPC has a destructive effect on cancer cells (OPC causes cancer cells to die and stimulates apoptosis), leaving healthy cells intact.

Black cumin oil / black seed oil

Black cumin (Nigella Sativa) is a plant that belongs to the ranunculus family.

In the Orient, black cumin has been used as a spice and as medicine for over 2000 years. In Asian countries, it is also known as black onion seed.

Characteristics

anti-inflammatory - pain-relieving effect- anti-allergic - antispasmodic - antibacterial - fungicidal - strengthens the immune system - lowers blood pressure and blood sugar - antioxidant - promotes digestion - anti-carcinogenic - migraine prophylaxis

Originally, black cumin was native to Iraq and Turkey. It also thrives in Southern Europe, India, Pakistan, and North Africa. Similarly, in the Islamic world, Prophet Muhammad's statement "In black cumin there is a cure for every disease except death" made black cumin very popular. Black cumin oil has been used successfully for centuries and is a staple in every household in the Middle East.

In naturopathy, it is used to treat the following complaints, among others:

allergies - neurodermatitis - psoriasis - to regulate the immune system - asthma - digestive problems - high blood pressure - migraine - cancer - inflammatory diseases

Black cumin oil is also used in veterinary medicine.

Another interesting fact is that studies published on the PubMed database show the proven efficacy against specific types of cancer.

Black cumin oil has also been proven to have a positive immunomodulatory effect in autoimmune diseases.

Possible side effects of black cumin oil
The strong concentration of the oil may cause mild stomach problems; exceeding the recommended dose may also cause irritation in the mucous membranes.

- 80 percent of all diseases are the result of an unhealthy diet
- **lack of exercise**, weak muscles, weak bones, low levels of mitochondria, no stamina
- **Micronutrient deficiency:** vitamin D, vitamin C, magnesium, selenium, zinc deficiency, etc.
- **Reasons for micronutrient deficiency:** medicines, unstable gut flora, monocultures, hybrids, pesticides, early harvesting, alcohol consumption, drugs
- **Acute trauma** - loss of loved ones, abuse, rape, bullying, etc.
- **Imbalance in mental state, the mind and soul** - stress and pressure at work, school, university or with family or friends, toxic relationships, bullying
- Environmental poisons/toxins - cigarettes, shisha, e-cigarettes, heavy metals, pesticides (glyphosate), aluminum in deodorant, pharmaceutical/hormone residues in tap water, fluoride in toothpaste, mercury fillings, preservatives, electrosmog (Wi-Fi, cell phone radiation), plastic, bisphenol A, synthetic detergents, estrogen-like chemicals, cosmetic products containing harmful substances (parabens, silicones, phthalates, etc.), vaccine ingredients (aluminum, foreign DNA, foreign proteins, antibiotics, polysorbate 80, formaldehyde).

More information on vaccinations can be found here:

Https://bachmair.org/index.php/english-consultation - https://www.vaccineinjury.info/ - www.vaccinefree.info

What makes us healthy or sick?!

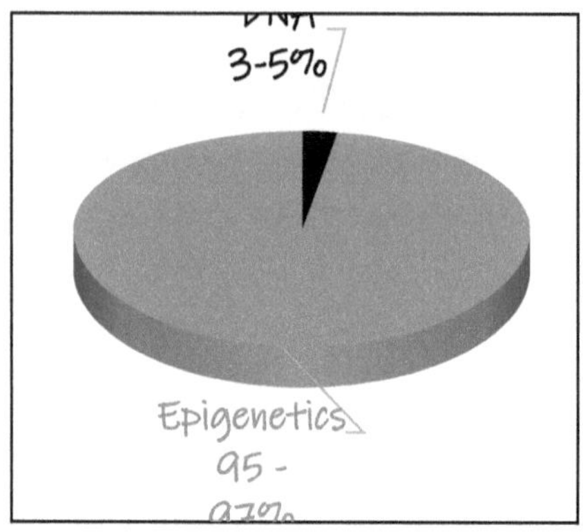

In most cases, it is not down to DNA.

Epigenetic Factors

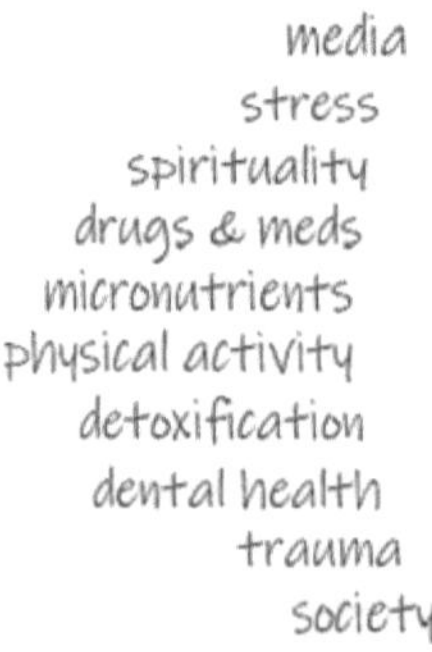
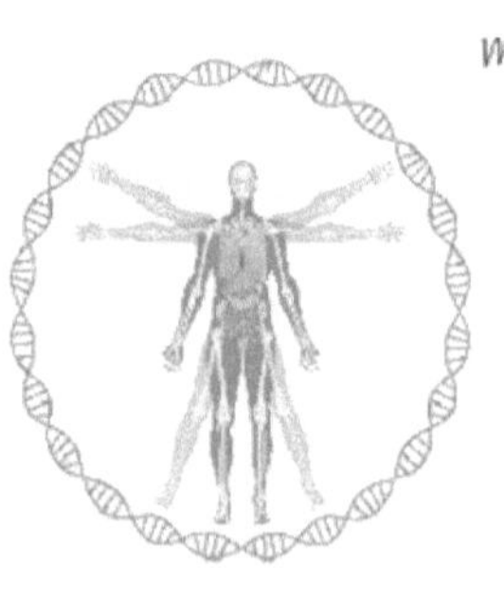

Mental health
meditation - autogenic training - neuro-linguistic programming - affirmations & autosuggestion - breathing techniques – psychoneuroimmunology therapy – scent and color therapy – outdoor walks – mindfulness mediation - reflection training - gratitude training - healthy sex life - healthy awareness of God

Healthy diet
food with oil/ protein (Budwig diet) - fasting - keto diet - vegan diet - vegetarian diet - paleo diet - Mediterranean food – natural spring water - reverse osmosis water

Naturopathy
orthomolecular medicine - Chinese medicine - detoxification - Ayurveda - fasting / intermittent fasting - environmental medicine (see Dr. Klinghardt or Dr. Mutter) - alternative medicine (see Dr. Rath) - vaccination injury treatment (see Andreas Bachmair)

Exercise
interval training - Nordic walking – core strength exercises - stretching - cycling - jogging - weight training (using your own body weight) - swimming - martial arts - ball sports - fascia training

For the mind and body
various massages - sauna - chiropractic - acupressure - infrared sauna - sunbathing – Kneipp cure hydrotherapy – activities that trigger oxytocin release

Electrosmog detoxification
set smartphone-free times in your day (or even an entire day) and replace these times with walks in the forest or in the great outdoors - Avoid smartphones when on vacation - Switch to flight mode at night - Switch off your Wi-Fi at night - Don't hold your smartphone to your head when telephoning and always keep it as far away from your body as possible.

The Conspiracy Theory

We are living in a time when much is distorted and does not appear as it really is. The media, influential institutions, and politicians all contribute to the mass of information we are inundated with every day. It is virtually impossible to follow the information paths anymore, and if you wish to understand things properly, you have no choice but to **take up journalism in your free time**. This is tedious and time-consuming, which is why many people chose not to do it, being busy as they are dealing with all the other distractions in life. When you get to the research stage, you'll end up online or will fill your time reading books on all manner of enlightening subject matter. You will start to have a different view on things and realize that there are all sorts of other opinions that stand in contrast to what mainstream media tells you. **As far as our cultural environment is concerned, especially the environment I grew up, skepticism has always been generally held to be a questioning attitude towards things.** Skepticism draws people closer to the reality of a thing because it allows them to look at things neutrally. Aristotle once said:

"Doubt is the beginning of wisdom."

In today's society, skepticism is more often than not associated with "conspiracy theories". We no longer have that "healthy dose" of skepticism. Any time you quote something that others are unfamiliar with or that doesn't fit into their world view, you are accused of being a conspiracist in order to silence you or portray you as someone who is going against the norm.

The following words by Soren Kierkegaard is a very fitting description of this state of affairs:

"The more people believe in one thing, the more likely it is that the view is wrong. People who are right are usually alone in their belief."

In most cases, skepticism and underlying doubt help us to take the more responsible and direct path. To use the words of Johann Wolfgang von Goethe:

Confident though you wish to feel,
I welcome the conflict within me.
For were it not for skepticism and doubt,
where would joyful certitude be.

Dear readers,
Maintain at all times a healthy dose of skepticism and

doubt, especially when it comes to your body and your mind.
For they are your most precious treasures!

Conclusion

By way of conclusion, I would like to thank you for taking the time to read my words. **It is not easy to negotiate your way through the jungle of information out there and distinguish right from wrong, especially in areas such as nutrition where there is no single version of the truth.** And this is precisely why I wrote this book. A book that you can use as a general guide to help improve your general well-being and enhance the quality of your everyday life. My intention was to show you an easy way to incorporate basic health and nutrition principles into your life. Throughout the years, these principles have helped me help others get on the path to better health. I hope that you, too, will benefit from this.

Thank you very much!

Yunus Güven

Acknowledgements

First and foremost, I would like to thank the Creator of the Universe and all those who participated in the creation of this book. I appreciate every minute of the hard work and effort you have invested in me, just to help me realize my dream of writing this book. You have become part of my biggest dreams. I hope we will change many lives for the better. The greatest heroes in my life deserve a special mention: my parents — for it is thanks to them that I have been able to pursue my passions and achieve such success. My parents have always encouraged my altruistic motives, my desire to work for the collective us, and taught me the importance of education and knowledge.

Mom and Dad - thank you for everything!

Last but not least: Thank you, Germany!
Thank you for affording me the privilege of receiving my education here, for allowing me to enjoy my education to the full to this day. Gaining an education in this country is not something I have ever taken for granted.

> Ingratitude is always a kind of weakness. I have never known men of ability to be ungrateful.
> Johann Wolfgang von Goethe

It is much easier for people to believe a lie that
they have heard a hundred times before than a
truth that is completely new to them.
Alfred Polgar

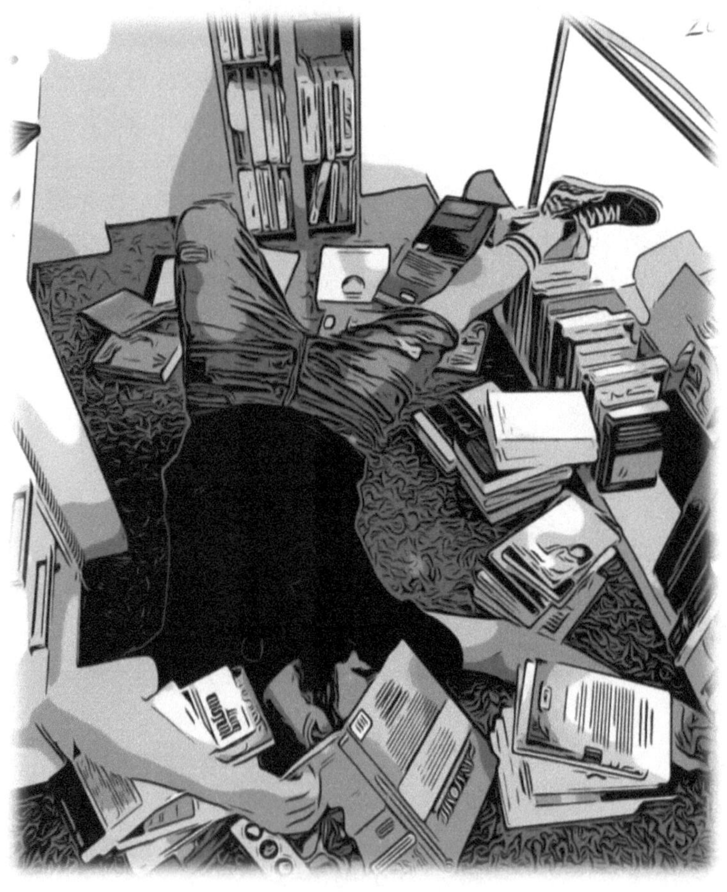

Anecdote about my addiction

Books are the reason I truly value having grown up in Germany. For in Germany, great value is assigned to knowledge and books.

Seeing how my fellow Germans connected with books, how much they valued books instilled in me the desire to ensure that books played a big role in my life.

Whenever I was invited to someone's house in Germany, all I could see was shelves full of books. Or when I was on the bus or train, people always had their noses stuck in books. When Germans bought a gift, it was always books .

Recording knowledge in books is a cornerstone of German culture, up to the point where laws are passed to protect and value knowledge, an example being fixed book prices.

And it is this cultural good that has become one of my deepest passions - books.

To quote Heinrich Heine:

"Of all the worlds that man has created, that of books is the most powerful."

Disclaimer

This book is a general guideline for a healthy lifestyle. Any suggestions made on health & nutrition behavior or preventative measures mentioned in this book are not intended to replace advice or treatment by qualified physicians, naturopaths, or alternative medical practitioners. Neither the author nor the publisher shall be liable for loss or damage to health arising from the use, both proper and improper, of the information contained in this book. The data and information presented here do not constitute health-related advertising statements on foods, biomaterials. or food supplements, but are a manifestation of my freedom of expression pursuant to Art. 5 | 1 of German Basic Law.

Bon Appétit!

Do you have any questions?

Interested in individual coaching?
Get in touch with me via Instagram - @the.dna.myth
or via email the.dna.myth@gmail.com

"The doctor of the future will give no medication but will interest his patients in the care of the human frame, in diet and in the cause and prevention of disease."
Thomas Edison (1847-1931)

Homework

Write 5-10 sentences about how valuable you and your family's health is to you:

____

____

____

____

____

____

____

____

____

____

____

____

____

____

____

____

____

____

____

____

Take a picture of your answers and send it to me on social media. Instagram: @the.dna.myth

What will happen if you fail to take responsibility for your health and have no interest in knowledge? Share your experience with me below.

____
____
____
____
____
____
____
____
____
____
____
____
____
____
____
____

Take a picture of your answers and send it to me on social media. Instagram: @the.dna.myth

If you've read the book, I would love to hear your thoughts.

____
____
____
____
____
____
____
____
____
____
____

Take a picture of your answers and send it to me on social media. Instagram: @the.dna.myth

How am I supposed to
make all of these changes
in my day to day life?

Take it slow! We all get
things wrong.
Asking "why" is what
matters most here.

"If we have our own 'why'
in life, we shall get along
with almost any 'how'."
- Nietzsche